Venipuncture for the Application of Blood Concentrates

VENIPUNCTURE *for the* APPLICATION *of* BLOOD CONCENTRATES

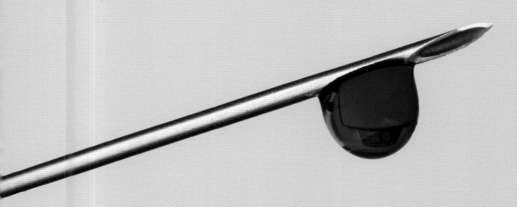

SHAHRAM GHANAATI, MD, DMD, PhD

Deputy Director and Chief Senior Physician
Department for Oral, Cranio-Maxillofacial and Facial Plastic Surgery
Johann Wolfgang Goethe University Frankfurt
Frankfurt, Germany

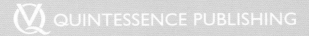 QUINTESSENCE PUBLISHING

Berlin | Chicago | Tokyo
Barcelona | London | Milan | Mexico City | Paris | Prague | Seoul | Warsaw
Beijing | Istanbul | Sao Paulo | Zagreb

One book, one tree: In support of reforestation world-wide and to address the climate crisis, for every book sold Quintessence Publishing will plant a tree (https://onetreeplanted.org/).

Library of Congress Control Number: 2023951176

A CIP record for this book is available from the British Library.
ISBN: 978-164724-1940

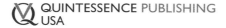

QUINTESSENCE PUBLISHING
USA

© 2024 Quintessence Publishing Co, Inc

Quintessence Publishing Co, Inc
411 N Raddant Road
Batavia, IL 60510
www.quintessence-publishing.com

5   4   3   2   1

Editor: Leah Huffman
Design: Sue Zubek
Production: Angelina Schmelter

Printed in the USA

CONTENTS

PREFACE

Blood collection and the preparation of blood concentrates is becoming more commonplace in the dental office. In this, as in every form of treatment, providing high-quality care is essential. Patient safety must be ensured, and the procedures used should be maximally efficient and effective. The foundation for this high level of care lies in the academic and nonacademic training of medical professionals.

With this goal in mind and based on extensive practical experience, I developed this textbook to empower dental professionals to perform blood collection and the preparation of blood concentrates safely, efficiently, and with the best possible results in the dental office. The book will teach you how to puncture a vein and draw blood step by step for the preparation of blood concentrates.

Although the highest priority has been placed on making the content practical and easy to follow, it is crucial to understand that only regular practice will bring the theory to life. Therefore, I strongly encourage you not only to read the procedures presented here but also to actively apply them in your dental office. With each blood draw and each preparation of blood concentrates, you will steadily improve your skills. Because medicine and dentistry are continuously evolving, it is all the more important to stay up to date to ensure the safety of your patients and the quality of your treatment results.

Acknowledgments

My sincere thanks go to all the participants in the Society for Blood Concentrates and Biomaterials (SBCB) beginners and user courses; without their valuable and active participation and the constructive exchanges that took place in these courses, this guide would not have been possible. I would also like to thank all the colleagues and founding and supporting members of the professional society, as well as the entire SBCB team, for their joint participation in this process. Our events to date were made possible to a considerable extent by their tireless and passionate efforts, which have helped the course participants achieve valuable learning experiences and success. Thank you as well to all those who have been open and patient in making changes and adjustments to this textbook to ensure that it will be a valuable guide for dentists and dental assistants to the world of blood collection and blood concentrates.

3D Animations

For better understanding of the content in this book, scan the QR code here to access 3D animations of each chapter with step-by-step description.

1

VENIPUNCTURE *and* BLOOD COLLECTION OUTSIDE *the* DENTAL CHAIR

Dentists and their practice teams are generally regarded as trustworthy, reliable, and extremely competent in their profession. After all, our professional training makes us experts in many areas, including periodontics, prosthodontics, and endodontics. Not only are we skilled in solving dental problems, but we are also able to keep our patients relatively free from pain and minimize the cosmetic issues associated with dentistry.

Nevertheless, for many patients, oral procedures can be an uncomfortable ordeal, and it is therefore important to build and maintain the patient's confidence. This is especially true when performing venipuncture and blood collection, because these procedures are unfamiliar to most patients in the context of dentistry and may give rise to doubt and skepticism. If the patient perceives any uncertainty in our eyes or facial expressions, they may judge it as incompetence, which can put a lasting strain on the clinician-patient relationship and leave the patient feeling uneasy about further treatment.

It is also important to consider the physical setup for the blood draw. A dental chair with an attached rinsing container leaves only one of the patient's arms available, which is not ideal (Fig 1-1). To avoid the awkwardness and limitations of the dental chair for blood collection, and to make the environment as comfortable as possible for the patient, blood collection is best performed in a different chair, but it must be in

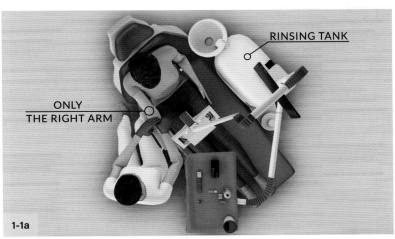

ONLY
THE RIGHT ARM

RINSING TANK

1-1a

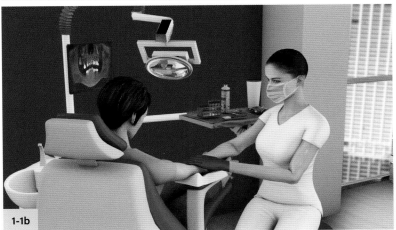

1-1b

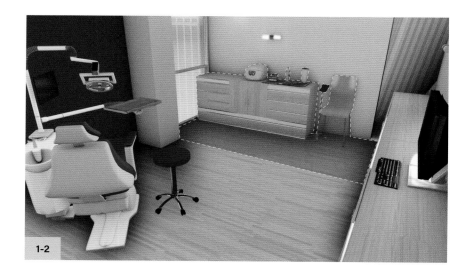

1-2

the same room (Fig 1-2). The chair should leave both of the patient's arms accessible, allowing venipuncture of the most visible and palpable vein.

> **IMPORTANT: The chair for blood draws must be in the same room as the dental chair to minimize the risk of mixing tubes from different patients, as the blood will go back into the patient's body.**

Once the workstation has been prepared (see chapter 2) and the patient is comfortably seated, place yourself on a mobile chair or stool and adjust its height to the arm to be punctured. This sitting position has a direct impact on the speed and efficiency of the procedure. Note that it is important for you and the patient to keep your legs together, as sitting directly in front of the patient with open legs may be experienced by the patient as uncomfortable or intrusive.

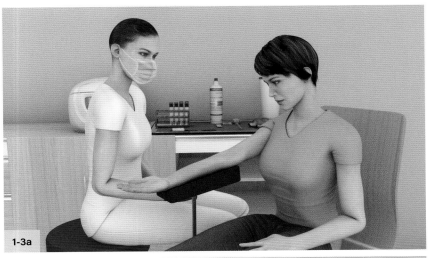

1-3a

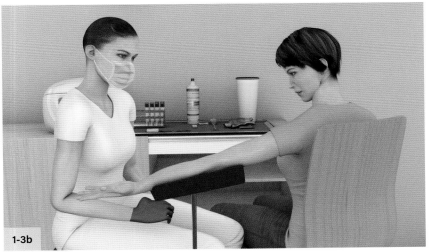

1-3b

If the patient's right arm is being punctured, you should sit with both legs to the left of the patient's legs (Fig 1-3a); if the patient's left arm is being punctured, you should sit with both legs to the right of the patient's legs (Fig 1-3b). To position the outstretched arm, it is recommended to use either a padded cushion or a mobile, height-adjustable arm support (see chapter 4).

2

ARMAMENTARIUM REQUIRED *for* VENIPUNCTURE

When preparing your workstation for venipuncture and blood collection, place all the materials you will need on a tray within easy reach of the chair where the venipuncture is to be performed. Unlike the area where the blood concentrates will later be processed, this workstation does NOT have to be sterile. The armamentarium is as follows (Fig 2-1, labeled accordingly):

1. Nonsterile gloves
2. Needle disposal box
3. Disinfectant spray or alcohol wipe
4. Butterfly needle
5. Tourniquet
6. Small sterile gauze pad
7. Adhesive bandage
8. Tube stand with red, white, and/or green tubes based on the centrifuge manufacturer
9. Centrifuge to prepare the blood concentrate

Before starting the blood collection, adhere an opened bandage to a nearby surface where you can retrieve it quickly (Fig 2-2). You will need this when you affix the butterfly needle immediately after the venipuncture.

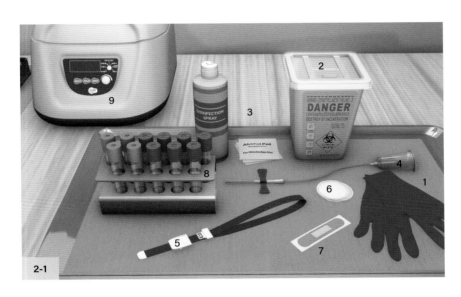

2-1

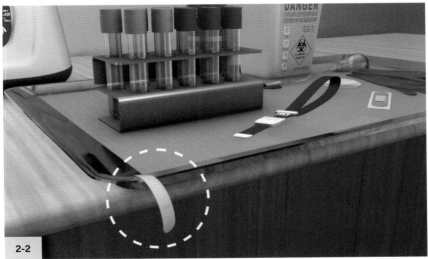

2-2

3

VEIN ANATOMY *of* *the* FOREARM

The forearm veins can vary significantly in their anatomy, with different patterns of connecting veins between the cephalic and basilic veins. The cephalic and basilic veins are often prominent and therefore lend themselves to venipuncture (Fig 3-1). If they are less prominent, the patient may have, for example, a relatively prominent median cubital vein (Fig 3-2).

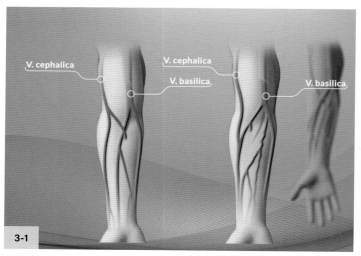

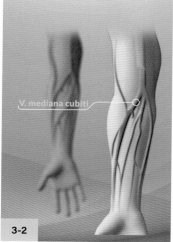

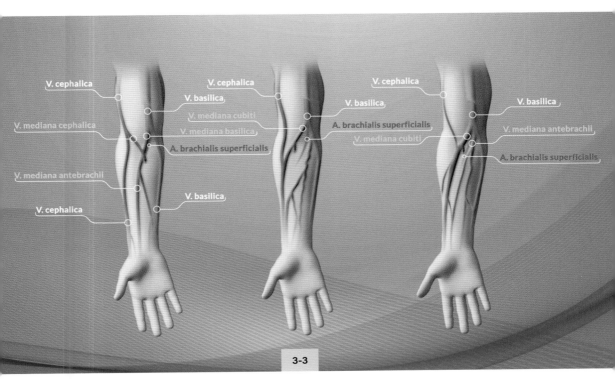

V. cephalica
V. basilica,
V. mediana cubiti
V. mediana basilica,
A. brachialis superficialis
V. mediana cephalica
V. mediana antebrachii
V. cephalica
V. basilica,

V. cephalica
V. basilica,
A. brachialis superficialis
V. mediana cubiti

V. cephalica
V. basilica,
V. mediana antebrachii,
A. brachialis superficialis,

3-3

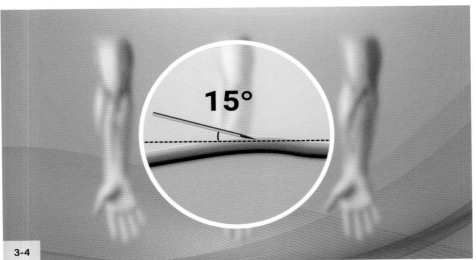

15°

3-4

Unlike the superficial brachial artery, the veins of the arm are located directly under the skin (Fig 3-3). That is why the needle should always be inserted into the vein at an angle of 15 degrees to the skin surface (Fig 3-4).

4

HOW *to* PLACE *and* ADJUST *the* TOURNIQUET

First, familiarize yourself with how to open and close the tourniquet before placing it on the patient's arm. The tourniquet has a relatively simple closure principle: It consists of a key element for insertion and a matching lock element (Fig 4-1). The latter has either a push button on the top or two side push buttons for unlocking or opening the tourniquet.

When you're ready to apply the tourniquet, hold it with both hands so that the key is on the medial side of the patient's arm while the lock is on the lateral side (Fig 4-2). Make sure the tourniquet band is not accidentally twisted. Approaching from below the elbow, apply the tourniquet four finger-widths above the cubital region (Fig 4-3) and lock it.

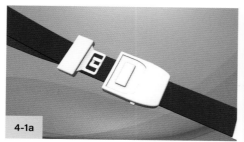

4-1a

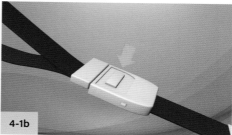

4-1b

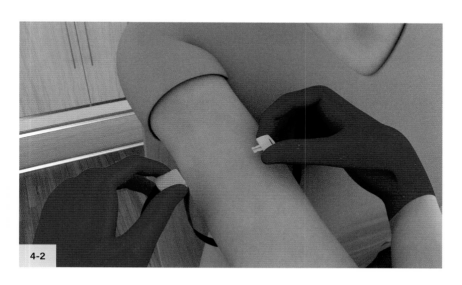

4-2

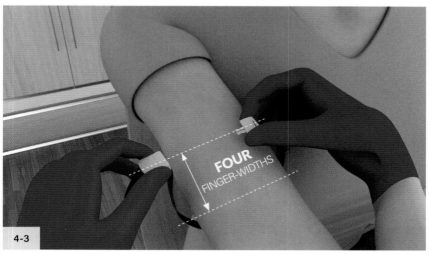

FOUR FINGER-WIDTHS

4-3

11

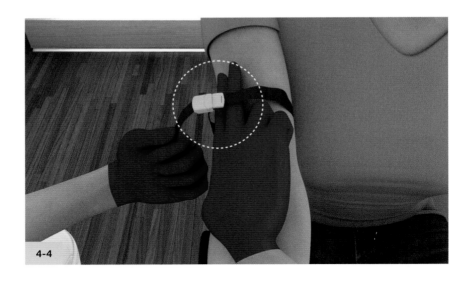

4-4

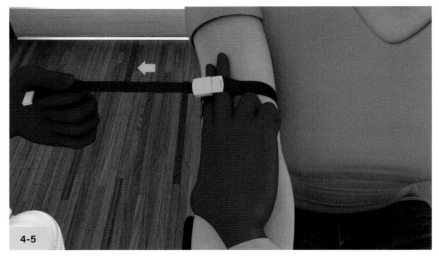

4-5

Using the hand that previously held the tourniquet key, place two fingers under the tourniquet (Fig 4-4). With the other hand, tighten the band (Fig 4-5) by pulling it away from the patient's body. The band is sufficiently tight when your two fingers underneath it feel significant resistance.

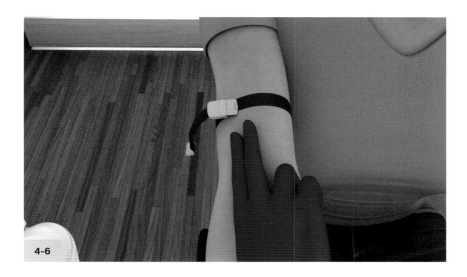

4-6

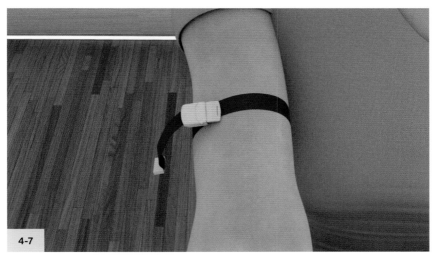

4-7

By using this method, you will achieve two objectives:

1. The patient's skin will not be bruised when the band is pulled.
2. The arterial blood flow into the arm will not be impeded.

Once the tourniquet is applied, pull your fingers out from under the band (Fig 4-6). The arm is now ready for venipuncture (Fig 4-7).

5

VISUALIZING *the* ARM VEINS

After the tourniquet has been correctly applied, make sure the patient's elbow is fully extended. If you are using an arm support, you can do this by adjusting its height (Fig 5-1). If you are using a padded cushion instead of an arm support, you can adjust the patient's seat height. The patient's arm should be in the most extended position possible.

You can now check the arm to see which veins are directly visible and palpable. To the touch, a vein has a slightly springy resistance. If you are unsure, it can be helpful to palpate the vein without gloves. Ask the patient to make a fist five times (Fig 5-2), or tap the cubital region of the patient's arm about five times with the hollow of your hand (Fig 5-3). This will release histamine, which will make the veins more visible (Fig 5-4).

Make sure the patient does not unintentionally rotate the arm around its longitudinal axis during the vein-detection process. This can result in the vein you previously located suddenly becoming invisible or no longer easily palpable. If you would like to additionally mark the vein that has been felt or identified, we recommend tracing the longitudinal axis of the vein to be punctured with a sterile pen after disinfecting the skin (see chapter 7).

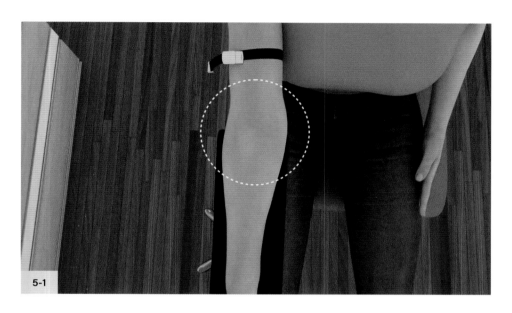

5-1

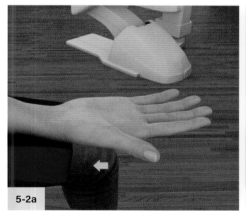

5-2a

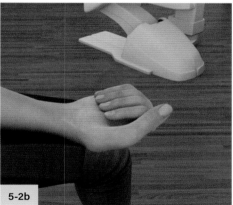

5-2b

15

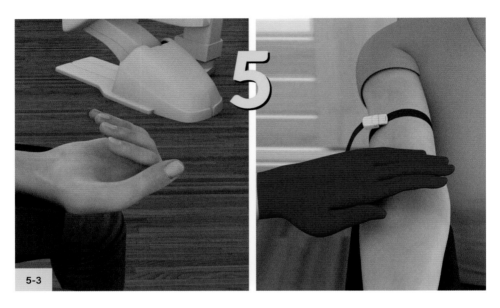

5-3

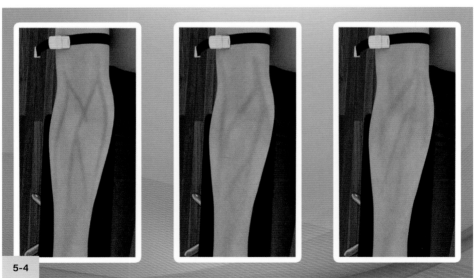

5-4

16

6

BUTTERFLY NEEDLES *for* BLOOD COLLECTION

The butterfly needle has two needle ends connected by a plastic line of tubing (Fig 6-1). One needle is for puncturing the vein, and it has a removable cylindrical protective sleeve (Fig 6-2). The other needle is for puncturing the collection tube so that blood can flow from the vein directly into the tube. This needle is covered by a nonremovable silicone sleeve (connector) that holds the collection tubes in place during blood collection (Figs 6-3 and 6-4). When you collect blood, make sure that the line connecting these two needles is not under tension or kinked.

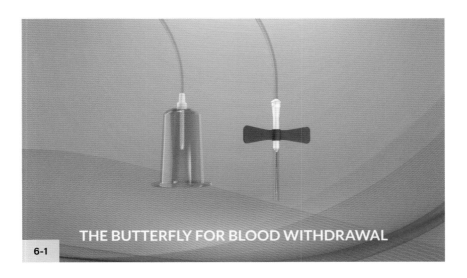

THE BUTTERFLY FOR BLOOD WITHDRAWAL

6-1

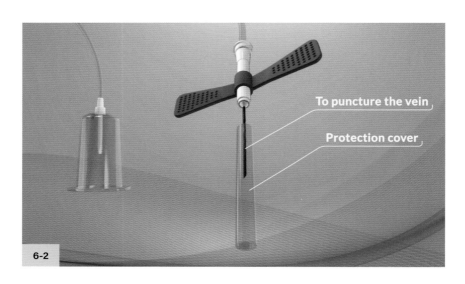

6-2

To puncture the vein

Protection cover

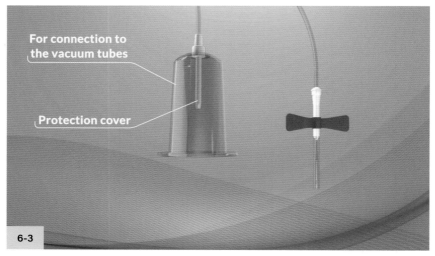

For connection to the vacuum tubes

Protection cover

6-3

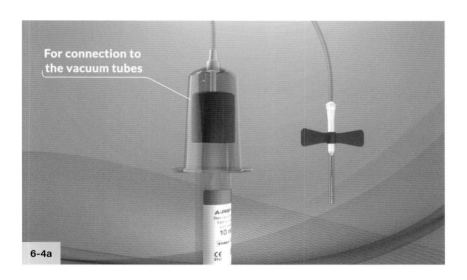

For connection to
the vacuum tubes

6-4a

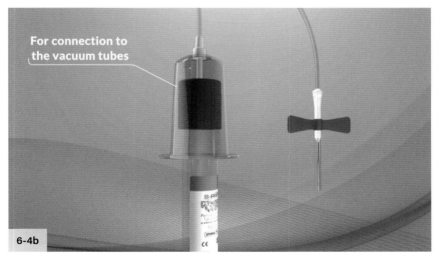

For connection to
the vacuum tubes

6-4b

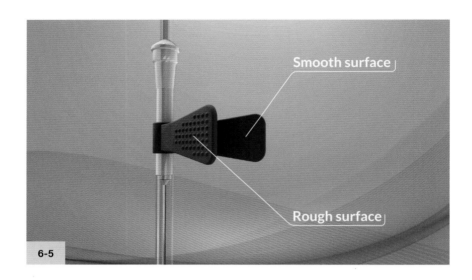

6-5

Smooth surface

Rough surface

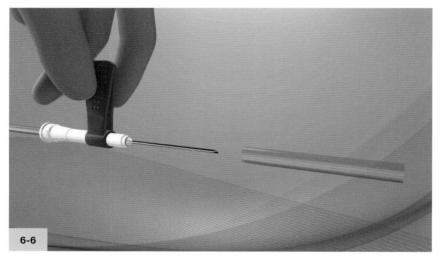

6-6

The butterfly wings have one rough surface and one smooth surface (Fig 6-5). You are holding the butterfly correctly if you can feel the rough side of the wing with your index finger and thumb (Fig 6-6).

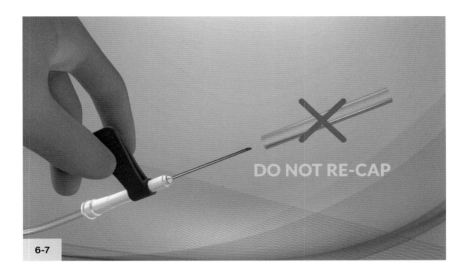

DO NOT RE-CAP

6-7

Only after all other preparations have been made for the venipuncture (see chapters 7 and 8) do you pick up the butterfly and remove the protective cap. Once you do this, you will see that the sharpened needle side is located below the needle opening. The butterfly is now ready for venipuncture.

It is important that the protective cover is NOT put back on the butterfly needle after completing venipuncture and blood collection due to the risk of injury and infection (Fig 6-7). Disposal takes place exclusively via the designated waste container (see chapter 2). Many butterfly needles have an integrated protective mechanism that pushes up a needle guard immediately after the puncture has been completed.

7

SKIN DISINFECTION
prior to
VENIPUNCTURE

Disinfecting the cubital region prior to blood collection is important to minimize the risk of infection. Be sure to wear medical gloves to prevent transmission of any microorganisms.

Hold the disinfectant spray approximately 20 cm away from the cubital region of the arm and spray twice (Fig 7-1). You can use your other hand to keep the spray mist localized to the cubital region and protect the patient's upper body and clothing from possible staining.

Using a piece of sterile gauze, wipe the sprayed area once from top to bottom (Fig 7-2), using sufficient pressure to remove any pathogens, then spray again and wait another 30 seconds to allow the disinfectant to air dry. It is important that the puncture site is as dry as possible before inserting the needle into the skin. Otherwise the alcohol in the disinfectant solution will cause a severe burning sensation in the skin around the puncture site. Do NOT wipe or touch the site again prior to venipuncture.

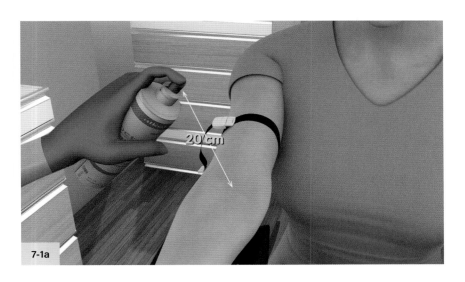

7-1a

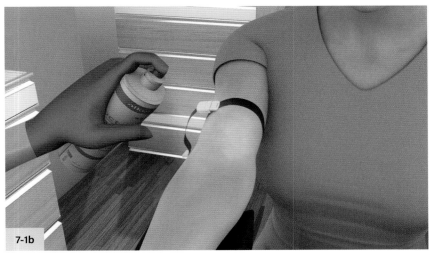

7-1b

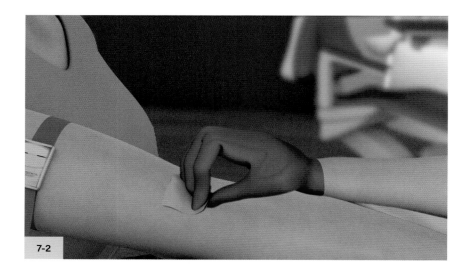

7-2

Alternatively, an alcohol wipe can be used to disinfect the skin. Again, be sure to let the alcohol dry completely prior to venipuncture to prevent any stinging.

8

TIGHTENING *the* SKIN *and* INSERTING *the* NEEDLE

Tightening the skin before venipuncture is an important step in making the veins easier to access and minimizing possible risks or delays in the process. It is not uncommon for cubital veins to roll under the unstretched skin of the arm, which makes venipuncture more difficult and unpredictable. The solution is to immobilize the veins under the skin. This is done by grasping the patient's arm, placing your thumb four finger-widths below the cubital region, and pulling the skin down in order to stretch it (Fig 8-1). Be careful not to apply excessive pressure; your goal is simply to stretch the skin and, by doing so, fix the target vein under the skin, facilitating easier access to it with the needle.

Successful venipuncture is performed as follows:

1. After removing the protective cap from the butterfly needle, grasp the upper half of the wings with your thumb and index finger (Fig 8-2). This allows you to keep an eye on the blood flow behind the wings while the blood draw is taking place. Be sure to hold the needle at an angle of about 15 degrees to the skin surface (Fig 8-3).

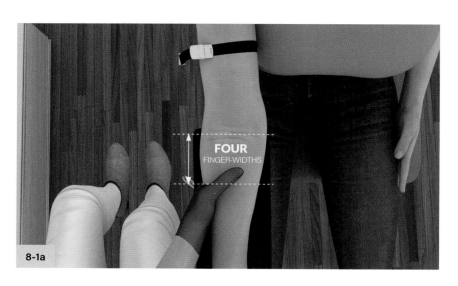

FOUR
FINGER-WIDTHS

8-1a

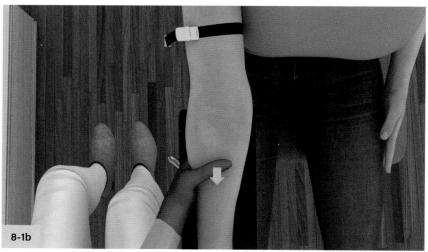

8-1b

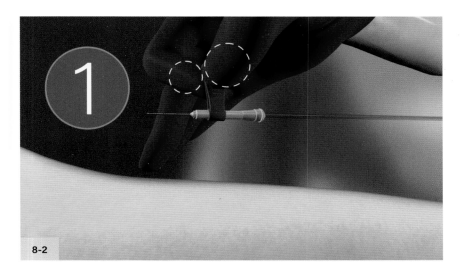

8-2

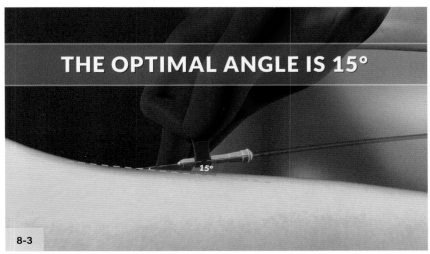

THE OPTIMAL ANGLE IS 15°

15°

8-3

2. Feel the longitudinal axis of the vein using the index and middle fingers of your other hand (Fig 8-4).

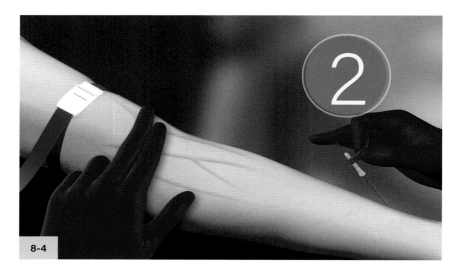

8-4

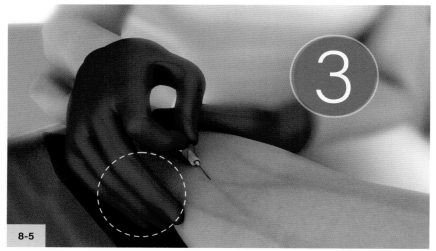

8-5

3. Stabilize the hand holding the butterfly. To do this, place your other three fingers on the patient's forearm (Fig 8-5). With your hand steadied in this way, you will more easily be able to align the needle with the longitudinal axis of the target vein.

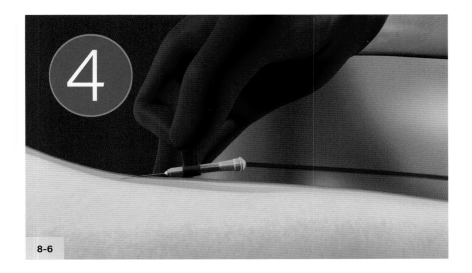

8-6

4. Now insert the needle quickly through the skin into the vein (Fig 8-6). The depth of insertion should be related to the dimension and prominence of the vein. The bigger the vein is, the more you can advance the needle inside. A minimum depth of 5 to 8 mm should be reached.

> Note: Act quickly and decisively. To minimize the pain the patient experiences, the needle should puncture the skin as quickly as possible, since it is only the contact between the needle and the skin surface that is painful.

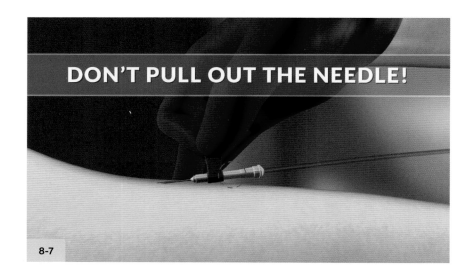

DON'T PULL OUT THE NEEDLE!

8-7

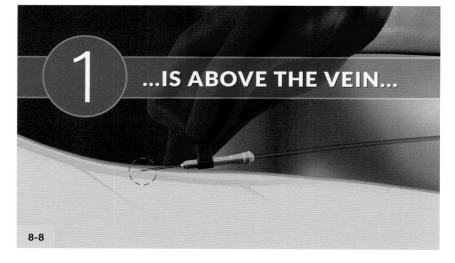

1 **...IS ABOVE THE VEIN...**

8-8

Once the needle is properly inserted inside the vein, attach a blood collection tube to the opposite end of the butterfly and hold it firmly until the tube is completely filled because of the vacuum inside.

If the needle is not inserted inside the vein correctly, do NOT pull it out (Fig 8-7). The needle could be above the vein (Fig 8-8),

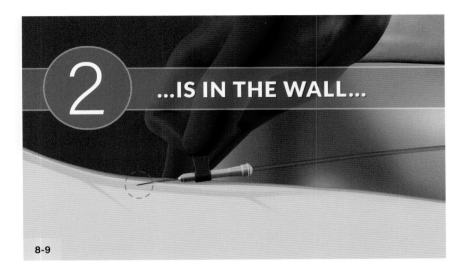

2 ...IS IN THE WALL...

8-9

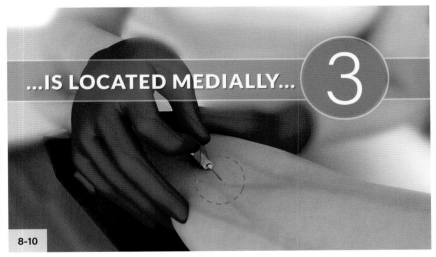

...IS LOCATED MEDIALLY... **3**

8-10

in the wall (Fig 8-9), or located medially (Fig 8-10) or laterally (Fig 8-11). **In all cases, keep calm and remain confident in what you are doing.** After you attach a blood collection tube to the other end of the butterfly, push the needle under the skin back and forth to reach the vein at the correct angle (Fig 8-12). Keep an eye on

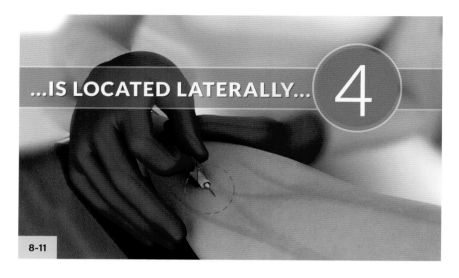

...IS LOCATED LATERALLY... 4

8-11

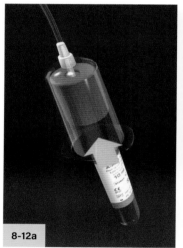

8-12a

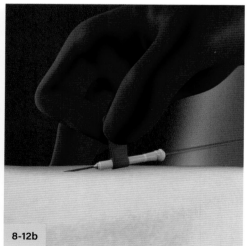

8-12b

the tube as you do this. With the needle inserted correctly in the target vein, the vacuum in the tube will draw the blood out, and you will see blood flow into the line behind the butterfly wings and then into the tube.

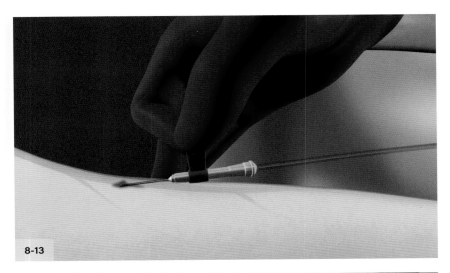

8-13

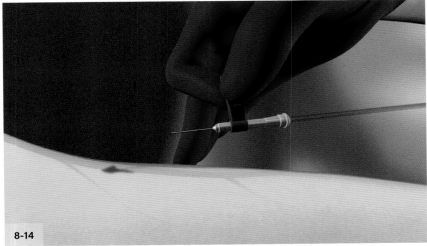

8-14

If a hematoma occurs due to a deep and incorrect puncture (Fig 8-13), loosen the tourniquet, remove the needle (Fig 8-14), and try venipuncture on the other arm.

9

FIXATION *of* the BUTTERFLY *to* the FOREARM SKIN

Once the vein has been punctured, ask your assistant or the patient to hold the butterfly tube in its position on the forearm with their index and middle fingers (Fig 9-1). Pressure on the butterfly tube should not be too firm, as that will interrupt the blood flow.

Do not remove the tourniquet until you have drawn the last tube of blood (Fig 9-2). Collection tubes for blood concentrates rely on a vacuum mechanism, and loosening or releasing the tourniquet may slow down the blood flow because the vein is no longer distended.

Now grab the bandage you stuck to the tray and use it to fix the butterfly tube to the skin of the forearm (Fig 9-3). If you notice that blood flow is decreasing or interrupted, adjust the position of the butterfly in the vein by repositioning the butterfly's wings. Once the bandage is correctly placed and blood flow is visible, the two fingers holding the butterfly tube can be released (Fig 9-4).

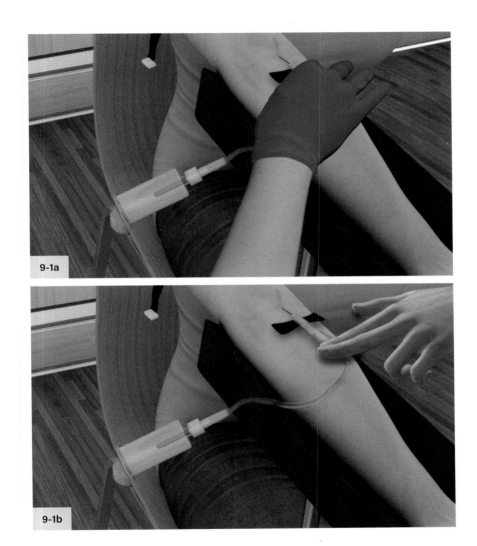

9-1a

9-1b

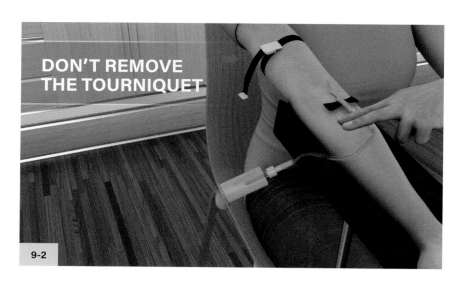

DON'T REMOVE THE TOURNIQUET

9-2

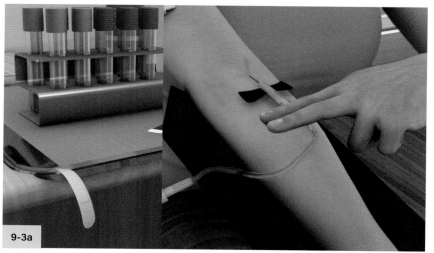

9-3a

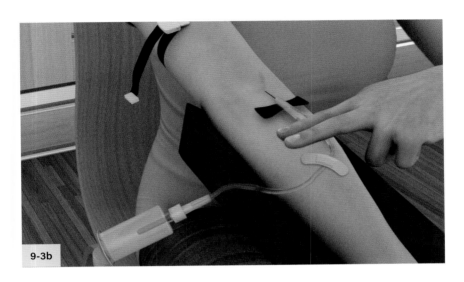

9-3b

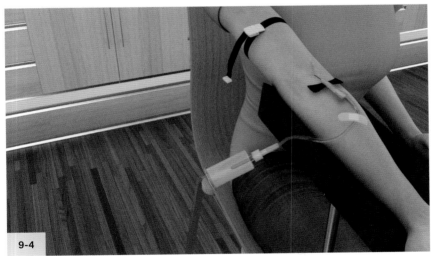

9-4

10

ATTACHMENT *of* GLASS *or* PLASTIC TUBES *to the* BUTTERFLY CONNECTOR

Take the butterfly connector in your dominant hand and a glass or plastic tube in your other hand (Fig 10-1). Insert the tube quickly and completely into the end of the butterfly connector (Fig 10-2; glass tubes shown in red and plastic tubes in green).

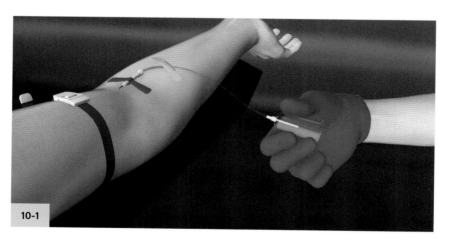

10-1

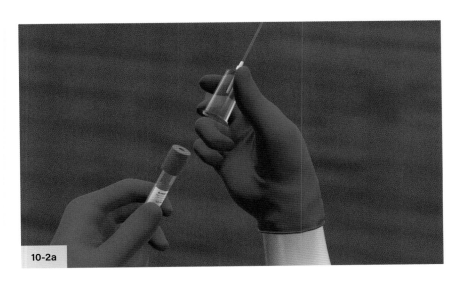

10-2a

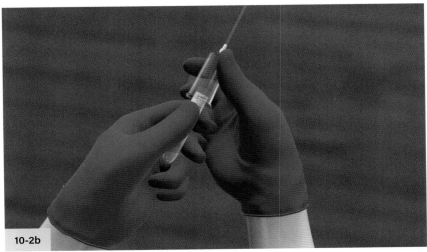

10-2b

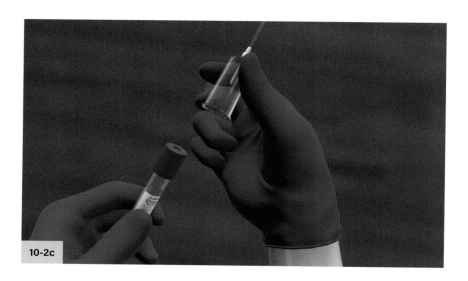

10-2c

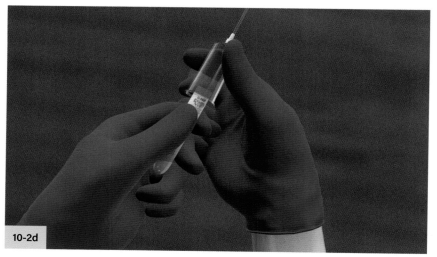

10-2d

Note: Once the tube is fully inserted into the connector, do not pull it back. If you do, you will lose the vacuum in the tube (Fig 10-3).

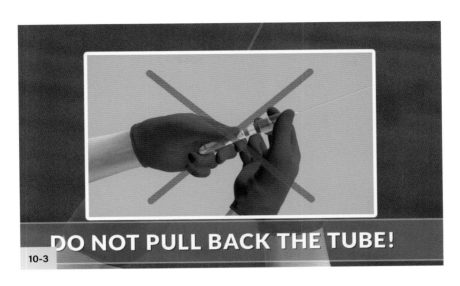

DO NOT PULL BACK THE TUBE!

10-3

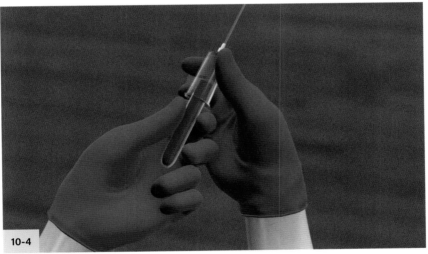

10-4

Turn the tube so that you can see the side not covered by the label. This way you can see whether blood is flowing into the tube and when it is completely filled (Fig 10-4). Keep the tube pressed tightly into the connector during the entire process.

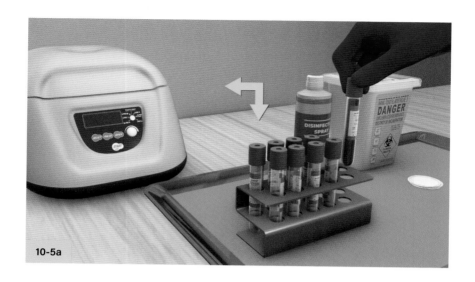

10-5a

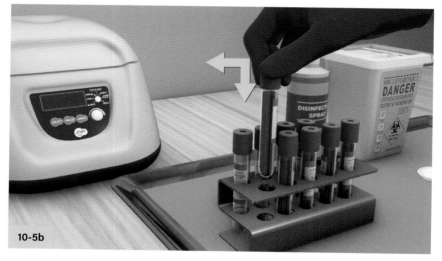

10-5b

When the tube is completely filled, remove it and place it in the tube rack or directly into the centrifuge (Fig 10-5).

11

REMOVAL *of* *the* TOURNIQUET *and* BUTTERFLY NEEDLE *from the* ARM

Once the blood collection is complete, unlock or open the tourniquet using **both hands** (Fig 11-1). This avoids the potential injury to the patient that can occur if the band snaps upon release and strikes the patient's chest area.

Ask your assistant or the patient to press on the butterfly tube with their index and middle fingers (Fig 11-2). Gently remove the bandage from the skin and reattach it to the collection tray nearby; you will use it again to cover the puncture site.

Carefully place a sterile gauze pad over the puncture site. Hold the gauze loosely over the needle while it is still in the skin (Fig 11-3). With your other hand, grasp the two wings of the butterfly needle and quickly remove it from the arm (Fig 11-4).

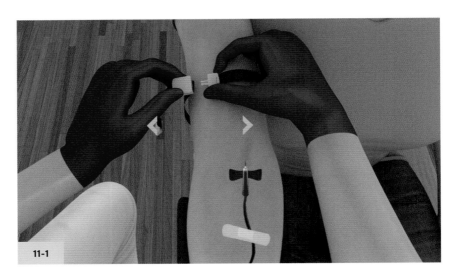

11-1

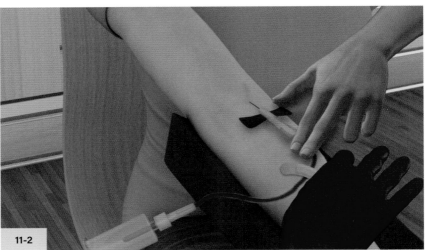

11-2

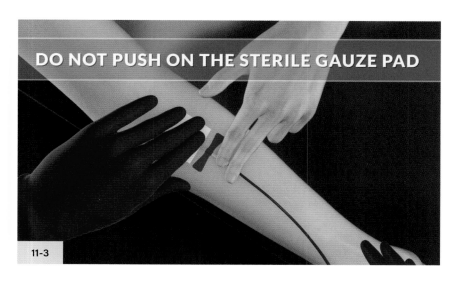

DO NOT PUSH ON THE STERILE GAUZE PAD

11-3

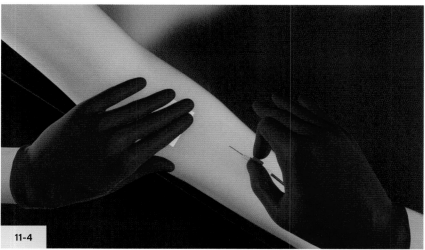

11-4

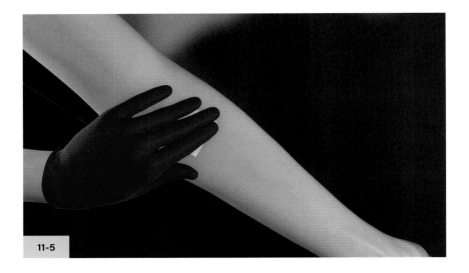

11-5

Due to the risk of injury and infection, do NOT put the protective cap back on the butterfly needle. Dispose of the butterfly needle immediately in the waste container.

Once the needle is removed, press down gently on the sterile gauze pad covering the puncture site (Fig 11-5). Do not push down on it.

Ask the patient to maintain gentle pressure on the gauze pad for about 5 minutes (Fig 11-6). As an alternative, you can ask the patient to flex their arm with the gauze compressed in the middle for 5 minutes (Fig 11-7). The patient can return to the treatment chair during this time.

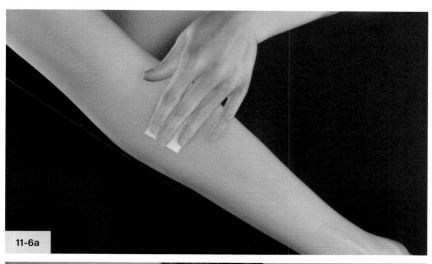

11-6a

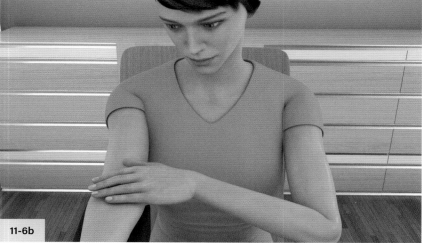

11-6b

47

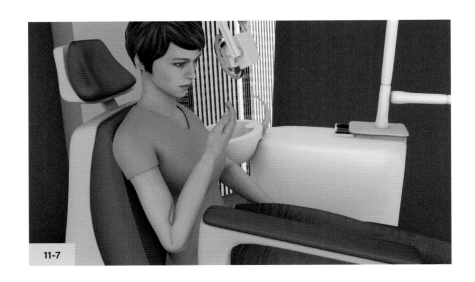

11-7

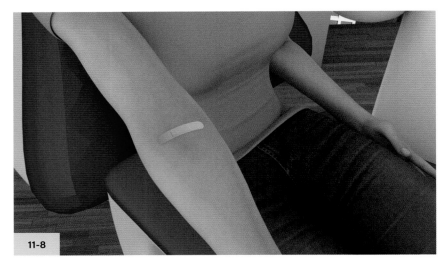

11-8

After 5 minutes, remove the gauze pad and apply the bandage to the puncture site (Fig 11-8).

12

HOW *to* BALANCE
the TUBES *within a*
CENTRIFUGE

Properly balancing a centrifuge is critical to ensuring accurate and reliable results when producing blood concentrates, no matter the model and manufacturer of the centrifuge. This chapter presents the options for correctly filling and balancing a centrifuge with 12 tube holders (Fig 12-1). Not all 12 tube holders need to be filled for the centrifuge to function correctly, but they must be filled in the following ways depending on how many tubes you plan to centrifuge.

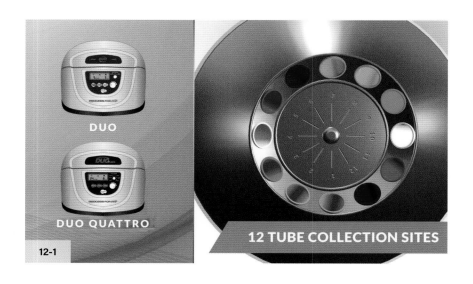

DUO

DUO QUATTRO

12-1

12 TUBE COLLECTION SITES

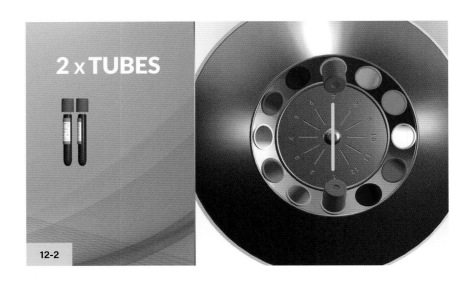

2 × TUBES

12-2

Two Tubes

When centrifuging only two tubes, place the tubes opposite each other in the tube holder of the same color (Fig 12-2).

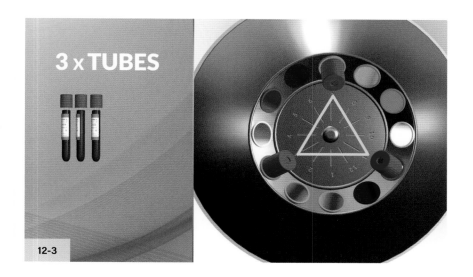

Three Tubes

When centrifuging three tubes, place the tubes in an equilateral triangle (Fig 12-3). You should primarily focus on the equilateral distance, not the colors of the tube holders.

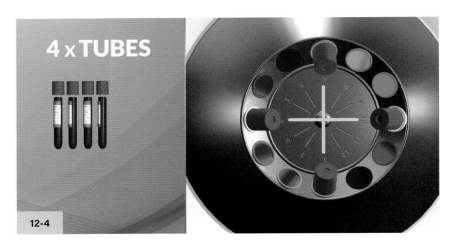

12-4

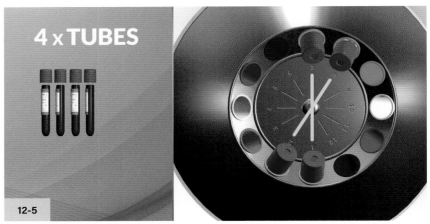

12-5

Four Tubes

When centrifuging four tubes, there are two options for achieving balance:

1. Place the four tubes opposite each other in the tube holders of the same color (Fig 12-4). In this scenario, there are gaps between the individual tubes.

2. Place a pair of tubes next to each other and the other pair opposite them (also next to each other) in tube holders of the same color (Fig 12-5). In this scenario, make sure that the tubes are in the tube holders of the same color.

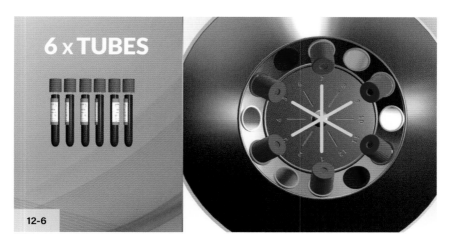

12-6

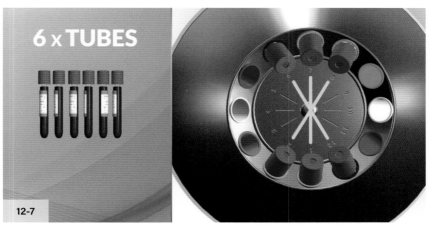

12-7

Six Tubes

When centrifuging six tubes, there are two options for achieving balance:

1. Place the tubes in every other tube holder (Fig 12-6).
2. Place three tubes together on one side of the centrifuge and three tubes opposite them (also together) in tube holders of the same color (Fig 12-7).

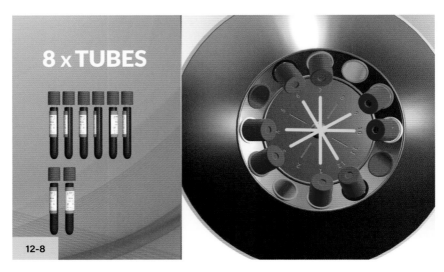

12-8

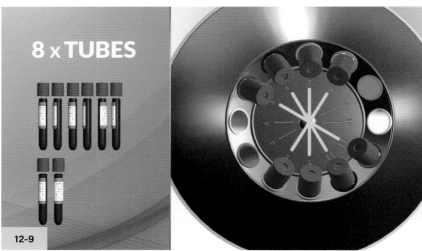

12-9

Eight Tubes

When centrifuging eight tubes, there are two options for achieving balance:

1. Place the tubes in pairs, with one tube holder free between each pair of tubes (Fig 12-8).
2. Place four tubes opposite each other in tube holders of the same color (Fig 12-9).

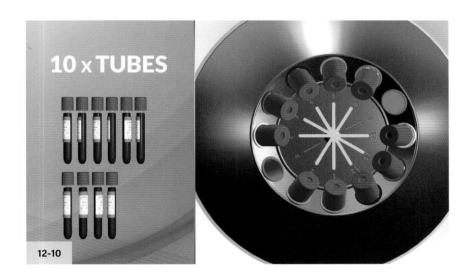

Ten Tubes

When centrifuging ten tubes, place five tubes next to each other and five tubes opposite them (Fig 12-10). One pair of tube holders of the same color will remain free.

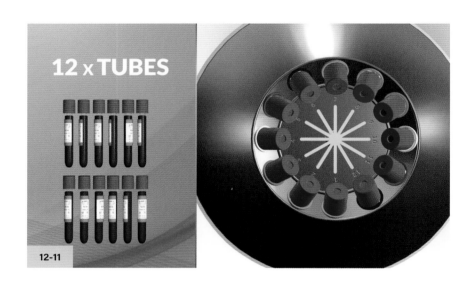

Twelve Tubes

When centrifuging 12 tubes, fill all tube holders (Fig 12-11).

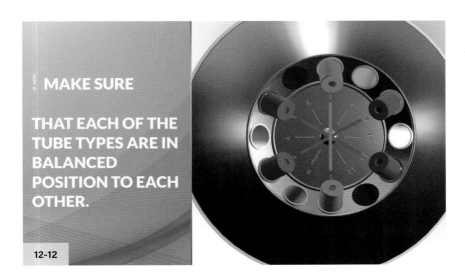

Important Considerations

If you are using both glass and plastic tubes, you must make sure that the centrifuge is balanced, with the glass tubes opposite each other and the plastic tubes similarly opposite each other (Fig 12-12).

If you do not have a counterpart for each tube—that is, if you do not have an even number of tubes or if you do not have an equal number of glass and plastic tubes—use a tube filled with saline as a substitute (Fig 12-13). Make sure that the substitute tube is plastic or glass according to what is necessary to balance the centrifuge. In fact, it is a good idea to have one glass tube and one plastic tube filled with saline or water prior to venipuncture in case you need it to balance the centrifuge.

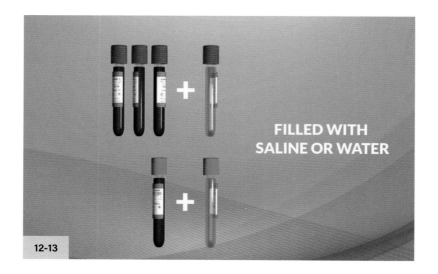

FILLED WITH
SALINE OR WATER

12-13

Once you have placed all tubes appropriately and set the specific protocol for duration and rotation speed, close the centrifuge lid and begin the centrifugation process.